HERBAL REMEDIES AND AROMATHERAPY FOR A RADIANT PREGNANCY

A Guide to Safe Practice, Holistic Care and Celebrating Your Unique Pregnancy Journey

KELLY WALTERHOUSE

TABLE OF CONTENT

Introduction

Pregnancy is a transformative journey, marked by numerous physical and emotional changes. In crafting this guide on herbal remedies and aromatherapy for pregnant women, the primary aim is to provide a comprehensive resource that empowers expectant mothers with natural tools to enhance their well-being. This book seeks to bridge the gap between traditional knowledge and modern approaches, offering insights into the safe and effective use of herbal remedies and aromatherapy during pregnancy.

Purpose of the Book

At the core of this book lies the intent to educate and empower pregnant women in making informed choices about their health and wellness. The purpose is not to replace medical advice but to complement it with holistic alternatives. By delving into the world of herbal remedies and aromatherapy, readers will gain valuable knowledge on harnessing the healing properties of plants and essential oils. The goal is to foster a sense of agency, allowing pregnant women to actively participate in their well-being and that of their unborn child.

Understanding the unique challenges and joys that pregnancy brings, this book aspires to be a trusted companion, offering guidance on incorporating herbal remedies and aromatherapy into daily life. From managing common discomforts to promoting emotional balance, each chapter is crafted with the purpose of enhancing the overall pregnancy experience through natural and nurturing means.

Importance of Herbal Remedies and Aromatherapy during Pregnancy

Herbal remedies and aromatherapy have a rich history of supporting health and well-being, and their relevance during pregnancy is profound. In this section, we explore why these natural approaches hold significance in the context of pregnancy.

Pregnancy is often accompanied by a myriad of discomforts, ranging from nausea and insomnia to anxiety and physical aches. While conventional medicine provides essential care, herbal remedies offer a complementary avenue that is gentle yet effective. The importance of herbal remedies lies in their potential to address these discomforts naturally, minimizing the need for pharmaceutical interventions that may carry unknown risks during pregnancy.

Aromatherapy, with its use of essential oils derived from plants, introduces a sensory and emotionally uplifting dimension to pregnancy wellness. The power of scents in influencing mood and relaxation is harnessed to alleviate stress, promote better sleep, and enhance overall emotional balance. Recognizing the psychological and emotional aspects of pregnancy, aromatherapy becomes a valuable tool in fostering a positive and harmonious experience.

Moreover, the importance of these natural approaches extends beyond symptom management. Herbal remedies and aromatherapy embrace a holistic philosophy that considers the interconnectedness of the body, mind, and spirit. This holistic approach aligns with the idea that supporting the overall well-being of the mother positively influences the developing baby. Through this book, readers will discover how herbal remedies and aromatherapy contribute to not only physical health but also emotional resilience and spiritual grounding during the transformative journey of pregnancy.

Safety Considerations

While the benefits of herbal remedies and aromatherapy during pregnancy are compelling, safety considerations take precedence. In this section, we emphasize the paramount importance of cautious and informed use of herbs and essential oils during this sensitive period.

Pregnancy introduces a unique set of considerations regarding the safety of any intervention, natural or otherwise. The book addresses the potential risks associated with certain herbs and essential oils, ensuring that readers are equipped with the knowledge to make choices that prioritize safety for both mother and baby. Safety guidelines regarding dosage, application methods, and potential interactions with conventional medications are thoroughly explored, empowering readers to navigate these natural therapies responsibly.

Furthermore, the book highlights the significance of consulting healthcare professionals before embarking on any herbal or aromatherapy regimen during pregnancy. Collaboration between traditional and medical approaches is encouraged to create a comprehensive and integrated healthcare strategy. By fostering a culture of safety and informed decision-making, this book aims to empower pregnant women with the confidence to embrace natural remedies responsibly, enhancing their well-being without compromising safety.

Understanding Pregnancy

Embarking on the journey of pregnancy involves a series of dynamic changes, both physical and emotional. This section aims to provide a comprehensive understanding of pregnancy, delving into the trimesters, developmental stages, common discomforts, and the comparative perspectives of traditional and herbal/aromatherapy approaches.

Trimesters and Developmental Stages

Pregnancy is typically divided into three trimesters, each spanning roughly three months and marked by distinct developmental stages. Understanding these stages is crucial for both expectant mothers and those seeking to support them through herbal remedies and aromatherapy.

First Trimester (Week 1-12): This initial phase is characterized by the formation of the embryo. While the body undergoes significant changes to accommodate the growing life within, common discomforts such as morning sickness and fatigue may arise. Herbal remedies like ginger tea can offer relief from nausea, while calming essential oils like lavender may help manage stress and promote relaxation.

Second Trimester (Week 13-26): As the baby's organs develop, the second trimester is often considered a more comfortable phase. However, expectant mothers might experience new challenges like back pain and hormonal fluctuations. Herbal remedies such as chamomile for relaxation and aromatherapy with uplifting scents like citrus oils can provide support during this period.

Third Trimester (Week 27-40): The final trimester sees the baby's rapid growth and the preparation of the body for childbirth. Common discomforts intensify, including swelling and sleep disturbances. Herbal solutions like nettle tea for nutrition and calming aromatherapy blends for better sleep become valuable tools in easing the challenges of this stage.

Understanding the nuances of each trimester allows for tailored approaches to herbal remedies and aromatherapy, addressing specific needs as they evolve throughout the pregnancy journey.

Common Discomforts During Pregnancy

Pregnancy, while a miraculous experience, often brings with it a range of discomforts. Herbal remedies and aromatherapy offer gentle alternatives to alleviate these common issues.

Morning Sickness: Nausea and vomiting, particularly in the first trimester, can be addressed with ginger tea or peppermint aromatherapy. The calming effects of these remedies can provide relief without the side effects associated with certain medications.

Back Pain: As the body adjusts to the growing baby, back pain is a prevalent discomfort. Herbal solutions like arnica for topical application and soothing aromatherapy massages with oils like eucalyptus or lavender can contribute to pain relief.

Insomnia: Sleep disturbances often accompany pregnancy, especially in the later stages. A calming herbal tea blend, incorporating chamomile and valerian root, along with a bedtime routine involving lavender essential oil, can promote better sleep.

Swelling and Edema: The third trimester may bring about swelling in the extremities. Herbal diuretics like dandelion tea, combined with gentle aromatherapy massages using anti-inflammatory oils such as chamomile or frankincense, can help manage swelling.

By addressing these discomforts with natural solutions, this book aims to empower pregnant women to navigate the challenges of pregnancy with a holistic and informed approach, minimizing reliance on pharmaceutical interventions.

Traditional Approaches vs. Herbal and Aromatherapy Solutions

Traditionally, diverse cultures have employed a range of practices to support pregnant women. This section explores the nuances of traditional approaches and compares them to the benefits offered by herbal remedies and aromatherapy.

Traditional Approaches:

Many traditional practices focus on dietary modifications, lifestyle adjustments, and the use of specific herbs. Practices like Ayurveda and Traditional Chinese Medicine emphasize balance in the body's energy or life force, known as Qi or Prana. These systems often incorporate herbal remedies, such as ginger and turmeric, to address various pregnancy-related concerns.

Herbal and Aromatherapy Solutions:

Herbal remedies and aromatherapy complement traditional approaches by providing additional tools for managing discomforts and promoting well-being. While traditional practices may emphasize dietary changes, herbal teas and infusions can offer concentrated sources of beneficial compounds. Aromatherapy, with its emphasis on scent and emotional well-being, introduces a unique dimension to the support available for pregnant women.

The key lies in integrating these approaches judiciously, considering individual needs and preferences. While traditional practices offer time-tested wisdom, herbal remedies and aromatherapy provide contemporary and accessible means to enhance the pregnancy experience. This book seeks to bridge these approaches, acknowledging the value in a holistic approach that draws from the strengths of both traditional wisdom and modern knowledge. By understanding the historical context of traditional practices and embracing the possibilities presented by herbal remedies and aromatherapy, pregnant women can cultivate a personalized approach to well-being that resonates with their unique journey.

Herbal Remedies during Pregnancy

Pregnancy is a time when the body undergoes significant changes, and the careful use of herbal remedies can provide natural support for both the mother and the developing baby. This section explores the world of herbal remedies during pregnancy, covering an overview of safe herbs, herbal teas, supplements and tinctures, and herbal infusions for common ailments.

Overview of Safe Herbs

Safety is paramount when considering herbal remedies during pregnancy. While some herbs are generally recognized as safe, others may pose risks. This section provides an overview of herbs that are considered safe for use during pregnancy.

Ginger (Zingiber officinale): Known for its anti-nausea properties, ginger is a go-to herb for alleviating morning sickness. Whether in the form of tea, ginger candies, or added to meals, it offers a gentle and effective solution.

Peppermint (Mentha × piperita): Peppermint is valued for its ability to ease indigestion and nausea. A soothing cup of peppermint tea can provide relief from digestive discomfort during pregnancy.

Chamomile (Matricaria chamomilla): Chamomile is often used to promote relaxation and alleviate anxiety. As a tea or added to a warm bath, it can be a calming ally for pregnant women dealing with stress.

Raspberry Leaf (Rubus idaeus): Raspberry leaf is renowned for its uterine-toning properties. Many midwives recommend it in the later stages of pregnancy to prepare the uterus for labor. However, it's advised to use it cautiously in the first trimester.

Nettle (Urtica dioica): Nettle is a nutrient-rich herb that can be beneficial during pregnancy. Its high mineral content makes it a valuable addition to herbal infusions for supporting overall health.

Lemon Balm (Melissa officinalis): Known for its calming effects, lemon balm can be incorporated into teas to help ease anxiety and promote relaxation during pregnancy.

While these herbs are generally considered safe, individual responses can vary. It's advisable for pregnant women to consult with a healthcare professional before incorporating new herbs into their routine, especially if there are pre-existing health conditions or concerns.

Herbal Teas for Pregnancy

Herbal teas offer a comforting and hydrating way to incorporate beneficial herbs into a pregnant woman's daily routine. This section explores specific herbal teas that cater to the unique needs of pregnancy.

Pregnancy-Safe Herbal Tea Blends:

Nausea Relief Tea: Combining ginger and peppermint, this tea can provide relief from morning sickness. It's gentle on the stomach and offers a soothing option for pregnant women dealing with nausea.

Uterine Tonic Tea: Incorporating raspberry leaf and nettle, this tea blend aims to support uterine health and prepare the body for labor. It's often recommended for consumption in the third trimester.

Calming Chamomile Tea: Chamomile's relaxing properties make it an excellent choice for a calming tea. This blend can be enjoyed in the evening to promote relaxation and ease stress.

Digestive Aid Tea: Fennel and ginger can be combined to create a tea that aids digestion and helps alleviate indigestion, a common discomfort during pregnancy.

It's essential to brew these teas in moderation and adhere to recommended guidelines. Pregnant women should avoid excessive intake of certain herbs, and if in doubt, consulting with a healthcare professional is advisable.

Herbal Supplements and Tinctures

In addition to teas, herbal supplements and tinctures provide concentrated forms of beneficial herbs. However, caution is required, and their use should be guided by healthcare professionals to ensure safety and appropriate dosage.

Calcium-Rich Herbal Supplements: Nettle and dandelion leaf supplements can provide an additional source of calcium, crucial for the development of the baby's bones and teeth. These supplements should complement a well-balanced diet.

Iron-Boosting Herbal Tinctures: Yellow dock and alfalfa tinctures are often used to boost iron levels naturally. Anemia is a common concern during pregnancy, and these herbal tinctures can be incorporated under the guidance of a healthcare provider.

Herbal Supplements for Nausea: For persistent nausea, supplements containing ginger or peppermint extracts may be considered. These can offer a concentrated dose of the nausea-relieving properties found in these herbs.

While herbal supplements and tinctures can be valuable additions, they should be approached with care. Dosages must be tailored to individual needs, and professional guidance is crucial to ensure their compatibility with the specific conditions of the pregnancy.

Herbal Infusions for Common Ailments

Herbal infusions involve steeping herbs in hot water for an extended period, extracting their medicinal properties. This method allows for a more concentrated preparation, offering potent solutions for common pregnancy-related issues.

Peppermint Infusion for Digestive Comfort: Peppermint leaves steeped in hot water can create a potent infusion that aids digestion and alleviates nausea. Sipping on peppermint infusion can be a pleasant way to address digestive discomfort.

Nettle and Raspberry Leaf Infusion for Nutrient Support: Combining nettle and raspberry leaf in a warm infusion provides a nutrient-rich beverage. This infusion can be particularly beneficial in supporting overall health and addressing nutritional needs during pregnancy.

Chamomile and Lavender Infusion for Relaxation: A blend of chamomile flowers and lavender buds steeped in hot water creates a calming infusion. This can be enjoyed before bedtime to promote relaxation and improve sleep quality.

Creating herbal infusions involves mindful preparation and attention to dosage. Pregnant women should be cautious about the strength of the infusion and the specific herbs used. It's advisable to start with mild infusions and gradually adjust based on individual responses.

In summary, herbal remedies during pregnancy offer a diverse range of solutions to address common discomforts and support overall well-being. From carefully chosen teas to supplements and potent infusions, the world of herbal remedies provides pregnant women with natural options to enhance their pregnancy experience. However, it is crucial to approach these remedies with caution, seeking professional advice to ensure safety and suitability for individual circumstances.

Aromatherapy for Pregnancy

Aromatherapy, the use of essential oils extracted from aromatic plants, holds immense potential in supporting the well-being of pregnant women. This section delves into the world of aromatherapy for pregnancy, covering essential oil safety guidelines, specific oils for calming and relaxation, addressing nausea and morning sickness, and soothing aches and pains.

Essential Oils Safety Guidelines

Before exploring the specific oils, it's crucial to establish safety guidelines to ensure the well-being of both the expectant mother and the developing baby.

Dilution: Essential oils are very concentrated and should be diluted before directly applying it to the skin. A general guideline is to mix 1–2 drops of essential oil with a carrier oil like almond or coconut oil.

Avoidance of Certain Oils: Some essential oils are best avoided during pregnancy due to their potential to stimulate contractions or cause adverse reactions. These include but are not limited to clary sage, basil, and rosemary. It's essential to research and consult with healthcare professionals to identify oils that may pose risks during pregnancy.

Ventilation: Ensure proper ventilation when using essential oils in a room or through diffusion. This helps prevent overwhelming concentrations of aroma and allows for a well-distributed and gentle fragrance.

Individual Sensitivities: Each individual may react differently to essential oils. Pregnant women should conduct a patch test before widespread use to check for any allergic reactions or sensitivities.

By adhering to these safety guidelines, pregnant women can enjoy the benefits of aromatherapy without compromising their safety or the safety of their unborn child.

Calming and Relaxing Oils

Pregnancy often brings about heightened stress levels and emotional fluctuations. Calming and relaxing essential oils can play a pivotal role in creating a soothing environment and promoting emotional well-being.

Lavender (Lavandula angustifolia): Widely known for its calming properties, lavender essential oil is a versatile choice for promoting relaxation. Its gentle aroma can help reduce anxiety and improve sleep quality, making it a valuable ally for pregnant women dealing with stress.

Chamomile (Matricaria chamomilla):
Chamomile essential oil, derived from the flowers of the chamomile plant, possesses relaxing properties. It can be used in aromatherapy to ease tension and create a serene atmosphere.

Ylang Ylang (Cananga odorata): With its sweet and floral scent, ylang-ylang essential oil is renowned for its ability to reduce stress and uplift mood. Its calming effects make it a beneficial choice for pregnant women seeking emotional balance.

Bergamot (Citrus bergamia): Bergamot essential oil, extracted from the peel of bergamot oranges, has both calming and uplifting qualities. Its citrusy aroma can help alleviate stress and promote a positive mindset.

Creating a blend of these oils in a diffuser or incorporating them into massage oils offers pregnant women a natural and pleasant way to enhance relaxation during this transformative period.

Oils for Nausea and Morning Sickness

Morning sickness is a common discomfort during the early stages of pregnancy. Aromatherapy can offer relief through specific essential oils known for their anti-nausea properties.

Ginger (Zingiber officinale): Ginger essential oil, derived from the root of the ginger plant, is celebrated for its anti-nausea effects. Inhaling the aroma of ginger oil or using it in a diffuser can help alleviate nausea and morning sickness.

Peppermint (Mentha piperita): Peppermint essential oil is known for its digestive benefits and can be effective in reducing nausea. Inhaling the scent or diluting it for topical application can provide relief during bouts of morning sickness.

Lemon (Citrus limon): The fresh and uplifting aroma of lemon essential oil can help combat nausea. Pregnant women can inhale the scent directly or add a few drops to a diffuser for a refreshing atmosphere.

These essential oils offer a natural alternative to pharmaceutical interventions for managing nausea during pregnancy. However, it's crucial to use them judiciously and seek professional advice if symptoms persist or worsen.

Oils for Soothing Aches and Pains

As the body undergoes physical changes during pregnancy, aches and pains are not uncommon. Aromatherapy can provide relief through essential oils with analgesic and anti-inflammatory properties.

Eucalyptus (Eucalyptus globulus): Eucalyptus essential oil is renowned for its ability to relieve respiratory issues, but it also possesses analgesic properties that can help soothe muscle aches. When used in a diffuser or diluted in a carrier oil for massage, it can contribute to pain relief.

Lavender (Lavandula angustifolia): Lavender, in addition to its calming properties, has mild analgesic effects. When applied topically through massage or added to a warm bath, it can help alleviate muscle tension and discomfort.

Frankincense (Boswellia serrata): Frankincense essential oil is known for its anti-inflammatory properties. Pregnant women can benefit from its soothing effects by diffusing it in a room or diluting it for topical application on areas experiencing pain.

Chamomile (Matricaria chamomilla): Chamomile essential oil's anti-inflammatory and calming qualities make it a suitable choice for soothing aches and pains. Incorporating it into massage oils or diffusing it in a room can provide relief.

By incorporating these essential oils into a holistic self-care routine, pregnant women can address physical discomforts naturally and create a nurturing environment that supports their well-being throughout the different stages of pregnancy. As always, consulting with healthcare professionals before incorporating new practices is advisable to ensure safety and individual compatibility.

DIY Remedies and Recipes

Pregnancy is a time when self-care takes center stage, and do-it-yourself (DIY) remedies offer a hands-on and personalized approach to nurturing well-being. This section delves into the world of DIY remedies and recipes, providing simple herbal solutions, aromatherapy blends for relaxation, and herbal infusions to boost energy and vitality during pregnancy.

Simple Herbal Remedies to Make at Home

Creating herbal remedies at home empowers pregnant women to tailor solutions to their specific needs, ensuring a personalized and effective approach to well-being. Here are some simple DIY herbal remedies:

Ginger and Lemon Tea for Nausea:
Ingredients:
- 1-inch piece of fresh ginger, sliced
- 1 tablespoon of fresh lemon juice
- 1 teaspoon of honey (optional)

Method:
1. Boil sliced ginger in water for 5–7 minutes.
2. Strain the ginger-infused water into a cup.
3. Add fresh lemon juice and honey if desired.
4. Sip slowly to ease nausea.

Calming Lavender Bath Salts:
Ingredients:
- 1 cup Epsom salts
- 10 drops lavender essential oil
- 1 tablespoon dried lavender flowers (optional)

Method:

    1. Mix Epsom salts with lavender essential oil.

    2. Add dried lavender flowers if using.

    3. Store in an airtight container.

    4. Add a few tablespoons to a warm bath for a relaxing soak.

Chamomile and Calendula Skin Balm:

Ingredients:

    - 1/2 cup chamomile-infused oil (infuse dried chamomile flowers in carrier oil)

    - 2 tablespoons calendula-infused oil (infuse dried calendula flowers in carrier oil)

    - 2 tablespoons beeswax pellets

Method:

    1. Melt beeswax in a double boiler.

    2. Add chamomile and calendula-infused oils.

    3. Stir until well combined.

    4. Pour into small jars and let it cool.

    5. Apply as a soothing balm for dry or irritated skin.

These DIY herbal remedies provide accessible and natural alternatives to store-bought products, allowing pregnant women to take charge of their well-being with ingredients often found in their kitchen or garden.

Aromatherapy Blends for Relaxation

Aromatherapy blends can be powerful tools for creating a calm and soothing atmosphere during pregnancy. Crafting personalized blends allows for tailoring scents to individual prefcrences. Here are a few aromatherapy blends for relaxation:

Serenity Blend:
- 3 drops lavender
- 2 drops chamomile
- 2 drops bergamot

Tranquil Sleep Blend:
- 3 drops lavender
- 2 drops frankincense

- 1 drop ylang-ylang

Stress Relief Blend:
  - 2 drops peppermint
  - 2 drops lemon
  - 2 drops eucalyptus

Uplifting Citrus Blend:
  - 3 drops orange
  - 2 drops grapefruit
  - 1 drop lemon

To use these blends, add the specified number of drops to a diffuser or mix them with a carrier oil for a calming massage. Adjust the ratios based on personal preferences and sensitivity to scents.

Herbal Infusions for Energy and Vitality

Pregnancy can sometimes bring about fatigue, and herbal infusions can be a delightful way to boost energy levels naturally. Here are a couple of herbal infusion recipes for energy and vitality:

Invigorating Herbal Infusion:**
   Ingredients:
   - 1 tablespoon dried nettle leaves
   - 1 tablespoon dried rosehip
   - 1 teaspoon dried peppermint
   - Method:
   1. Place herbs in a teapot or infuser.
   2. Pour hot water over the herbs.
   3. Steep for 5–7 minutes.
   4. Strain and enjoy.

Energizing Citrus Infusion:
   Ingredients:
   - 1 tablespoon dried lemon balm
   - 1 tablespoon dried lemongrass

- 1 teaspoon dried ginger
- Method:
    1. Combine herbs in a teapot or infuser.
    2. Pour hot water over the herbs.
    3. Steep for 5–7 minutes.
    4. Strain and savor the revitalizing infusion.

These herbal infusions not only provide a natural energy boost but also contribute to hydration, an essential aspect of maintaining vitality during pregnancy.

Incorporating these DIY remedies and recipes into a daily routine allows pregnant women to actively engage in self-care, fostering a sense of well-being and empowerment. However, it's essential to be mindful of individual sensitivities and consult with healthcare professionals, especially when introducing new ingredients or practices during pregnancy.

Nutrition and Wellness

Pregnancy is a transformative period that demands special attention to nutrition and overall wellness. This section explores the crucial connection between nutrition and wellness during pregnancy, emphasizing the importance of balanced nutrition, incorporating herbs into a healthy pregnancy diet, and identifying superfoods that contribute to the well-being of both the mother and the developing baby.

Importance of Balanced Nutrition

Balanced nutrition is the cornerstone of a healthy pregnancy. The body undergoes numerous changes to support the growing baby, making it imperative to provide essential nutrients for optimal development. Here are key components highlighting the importance of balanced nutrition during pregnancy:

Fetal Development: Proper nutrition is essential for the development of the baby's organs, tissues, and overall growth. Adequate intake of nutrients like folate, iron, calcium, and essential fatty acids is crucial during different stages of pregnancy.

Maternal Health: Maintaining balanced nutrition is equally vital for the health of the expectant mother. A well-nourished body can better cope with the physical demands of pregnancy, reduce the risk of complications, and support the mother's overall well-being.

Energy and Stamina: Pregnancy often brings about increased fatigue and energy demands. A balanced diet ensures an adequate supply of energy, vitamins, and minerals, contributing to sustained stamina and vitality throughout the pregnancy.

Immune Support: Proper nutrition plays a role in supporting the immune system, helping to protect both the mother and the developing baby from infections and illnesses.

Blood Sugar Regulation: Balancing blood sugar levels becomes especially important during pregnancy. A diet rich in complex carbohydrates, fiber, and balanced protein helps regulate blood sugar and reduces the risk of gestational diabetes.

Incorporating a variety of nutrient-dense foods, including fruits, vegetables, whole grains, lean proteins, and dairy products, contributes to a well-rounded and balanced diet essential for a healthy pregnancy.

Incorporating Herbs into a Healthy Pregnancy Diet

Herbs can be valuable additions to a healthy pregnancy diet, providing flavor, nutrients, and potential therapeutic benefits. Here are some ways to incorporate herbs into meals during pregnancy:

Fresh Herbs in Cooking: Adding fresh herbs like basil, parsley, dill, and cilantro to meals not only enhances flavor but also introduces additional vitamins and minerals. These herbs can be sprinkled over salads, incorporated into sauces, or used as garnishes for various dishes.

Herbal Infusions and Teas: Nettle, red raspberry leaf, and peppermint are examples of herbs that can be consumed as infusions or teas. These herbal beverages not only contribute to hydration but also offer nutritional benefits. However, pregnant women should exercise caution and limit the intake of certain herbs, especially in concentrated forms.

Herb-Infused Oils and Vinegars: Creating herb-infused oils or vinegars is a simple way to introduce herbal flavors into meals. Rosemary-infused olive oil or tarragon-infused vinegar can add a delightful twist to salads and various dishes.

Herbal Seasoning Blends: Combining dried herbs like thyme, oregano, and sage can create versatile herbal seasoning blends. These blends can be used to season meats, vegetables, and other dishes, enhancing both taste and nutritional content.

It's essential to exercise caution and moderation when incorporating herbs into the diet, as some herbs may have contraindications during pregnancy. Consulting with healthcare professionals and being mindful of individual sensitivities is advisable.

Superfoods for Pregnancy

Superfoods are nutrient-dense foods that provide a wealth of vitamins, minerals, and antioxidants. Incorporating these superfoods into a pregnancy diet can offer a range of health benefits. Here are some superfoods particularly beneficial during pregnancy:

1. Leafy Greens: Spinach, kale, and Swiss chard are rich in folate, iron, and calcium. These nutrients are crucial for fetal development and can help prevent anemia during pregnancy.

2. Berries: Blueberries, strawberries, and raspberries are packed with antioxidants, vitamin C, and fiber. These fruits contribute to a healthy immune system and support digestion.

3. Avocado: Avocado is a nutrient powerhouse, providing healthy fats, potassium, and folate. The monounsaturated fats in avocados support the development of the baby's brain and nervous system.

4. Greek Yogurt: Greek yogurt is an excellent source of protein, calcium, and probiotics. It supports bone health, digestive function, and provides a protein boost important for maternal and fetal tissues.

5. Quinoa: Quinoa is a versatile whole grain that provides a complete protein source, essential amino acids, and fiber. It contributes to maintaining stable blood sugar levels and supports overall energy.

6. Chia Seeds: Chia seeds are rich in omega-3 fatty acids, fiber, and minerals. They support brain development in the baby and contribute to digestive health.

7. Salmon: Fatty fish like salmon are high in omega-3 fatty acids, which are crucial for the development of the baby's brain and eyes. Salmon also provides high-quality protein and vitamin D.

8. Eggs: Eggs are a nutrient-dense source of protein, choline, and various vitamins and minerals. Choline is essential for fetal brain development.

9. Lentils: Lentils are an excellent plant-based source of protein, iron, and folate. They contribute to preventing iron-deficiency anemia and support overall maternal health.

10. Sweet Potatoes: Sweet potatoes are rich in beta-carotene, which is converted into vitamin A in the body. Vitamin A is essential for fetal development and supports immune function.

Incorporating these superfoods into meals and snacks during pregnancy provides a diverse range of nutrients that contribute to the health and vitality of both the mother and the developing baby.

In conclusion, focusing on balanced nutrition and overall wellness is paramount during pregnancy. A diet rich in a variety of nutrient-dense foods, including superfoods and thoughtfully chosen herbs, supports the unique needs of this transformative period. By adopting a mindful and individualized approach to nutrition, pregnant women can optimize their well-being and contribute to the healthy development of their unborn child. As always, consulting with healthcare professionals for personalized guidance is essential to ensure the safety and appropriateness of dietary choices during pregnancy.

51 Herbal Remedies And Aromatherapy For A Radiant Pregnancy

Exercise and Self-Care

Pregnancy is a time when maintaining physical and emotional well-being is crucial. This section explores the role of exercise and self-care during pregnancy, providing insights into gentle exercises tailored for pregnant women, incorporating aromatherapy into self-care routines, and effective stress reduction techniques to promote overall health and balance.

Gentle Exercises for Pregnant Women

Staying active during pregnancy offers a myriad of benefits, including improved mood, increased stamina, and better overall health. However, it's important to choose exercises that are gentle and safe for both the expectant mother and the developing baby. Here are some recommended gentle exercises for pregnant women:

1. Prenatal Yoga: Prenatal yoga focuses on gentle stretches, controlled breathing, and relaxation. It helps improve flexibility, balance, and can alleviate common pregnancy discomforts.

2. Walking: A low-impact and accessible exercise, walking supports cardiovascular health and can be adapted to various fitness levels. It also provides an opportunity for fresh air and gentle movement.

3. Swimming: Swimming and water aerobics are excellent choices for pregnant women. Buoyancy in the water reduces impact on joints, and the resistance of the water enhances muscle tone.

4. Prenatal Pilates: Prenatal Pilates emphasizes core strength, flexibility, and posture. Modified exercises are designed to accommodate the changing body of a pregnant woman while promoting overall fitness.

5. Stationary Cycling: Using a stationary bike provides a low-impact cardiovascular workout. Adjusting the resistance allows for customization based on individual fitness levels.

6. Prenatal Dance: Dance classes designed for pregnant women incorporate movements that support flexibility and cardiovascular health. It's an enjoyable way to stay active and connect with other expectant mothers.

7. Strength Training with Modifications: Incorporating light weights or resistance bands can help maintain muscle tone. However, it's essential to use proper form and opt for lower resistance, focusing on higher repetitions.

8. Pelvic Floor Exercises (Kegels): Strengthening the pelvic floor muscles can be beneficial during pregnancy and may assist in preparation for labor. Kegel exercises involve contracting and relaxing the pelvic muscles.

Before engaging in any exercise routine during pregnancy, it's crucial to consult with a healthcare provider. They can provide personalized advice based on individual health conditions and the specific needs of the pregnancy.

Incorporating Aromatherapy into Self-Care Routines

Self-care during pregnancy involves nurturing the mind, body, and spirit. Aromatherapy, the use of essential oils, can be a delightful addition to self-care routines, providing a sensory experience that supports relaxation and emotional well-being.

1. Aromatherapy Massage: Diluting essential oils in a carrier oil and incorporating them into a gentle massage routine can promote relaxation and alleviate muscle tension. Oils like lavender, chamomile, and frankincense are popular choices for their calming effects.

2. Relaxing Bath with Essential Oils: Adding a few drops of pregnancy-safe essential oils to a warm bath creates a soothing experience. Scents like lavender, ylang-ylang, and citrus oils can enhance relaxation and provide a moment of tranquility.

3. Aromatherapy Diffusion: Using an essential oil diffuser in the home allows for the continuous release of aromatic molecules into the air. Diffusing calming oils like bergamot, cedarwood, or geranium can create a peaceful environment.

4. Scented Pillows or Sachets: Placing a small pillow or sachet infused with calming essential oils near the sleeping area can enhance the quality of sleep. Lavender and chamomile are popular choices for their sleep-inducing properties.

5. DIY Aromatherapy Blends: Experimenting with personalized aromatherapy blends allows pregnant women to tailor scents to their preferences. Blends like lavender and vanilla or citrus and mint can create uplifting and refreshing atmospheres.

It's important to follow safety guidelines when using essential oils during pregnancy. Dilution, moderation, and avoidance of certain oils should be considered. Pregnant women should consult with healthcare professionals if they have any concerns about the use of essential oils.

Stress Reduction Techniques

Stress reduction is a vital aspect of self-care during pregnancy. Elevated stress levels can impact both maternal and fetal well-being. Here are effective stress reduction techniques for expectant mothers:

1. Mindful Breathing: Practicing mindful breathing exercises, such as deep belly breathing or diaphragmatic breathing, can activate the body's relaxation response. This helps reduce stress and promotes a sense of calm.

2. Meditation: Incorporating mindfulness meditation into daily routines allows pregnant women to cultivate a focused and present state of mind. Guided meditations tailored for pregnancy can address specific concerns and promote relaxation.

3. Gentle Stretching: Incorporating gentle stretching exercises, such as those found in prenatal yoga, can release tension from the body and contribute to a sense of physical well-being.

4. Journaling: Writing down thoughts and feelings in a journal can be a therapeutic way to process emotions. Reflecting on positive aspects of the pregnancy journey can shift focus away from stressors.

5. Connecting with Nature: Spending time outdoors, whether it's a leisurely walk in a park or simply sitting in a garden, provides a natural environment that supports relaxation and stress reduction.

6. Visualization: Engaging in visualization exercises where expectant mothers imagine peaceful scenes or positive outcomes can be a powerful tool for reducing stress and promoting a positive mindset.

7. Gentle Exercise: As mentioned earlier, activities like walking, swimming, or prenatal yoga not only contribute to physical health but also release endorphins, which are natural stress relievers.

8. Support Networks:
Maintaining connections with supportive friends, family, or fellow expectant mothers can offer emotional support and a sense of community.

Combining these stress reduction techniques with exercise, aromatherapy, and other self-care practices creates a holistic approach to well-being during pregnancy. As always, it's important to communicate with healthcare professionals to ensure that chosen techniques align with individual health conditions and the specific needs of the pregnancy.

Exercise and self-care play integral roles in promoting overall health and well-being during pregnancy. Gentle exercises tailored for expectant mothers contribute to physical fitness, while self-care practices such as aromatherapy and stress reduction techniques nurture emotional and mental well-being. By embracing a holistic approach to self-care, pregnant women can navigate the transformative journey of pregnancy with resilience and a sense of balance.

61 Herbal Remedies And Aromatherapy For A Radiant Pregnancy

Consulting with Healthcare Professionals

Pregnancy is a complex and unique journey for each woman, and seeking guidance from healthcare professionals is paramount for a safe and healthy experience. This section emphasizes the importance of consulting with healthcare professionals during pregnancy, outlining when to seek professional advice and providing insights into integrating herbal remedies and aromatherapy with medical care.

When to Seek Professional Advice

Navigating the myriad of changes and challenges during pregnancy requires a collaborative approach between expectant mothers and their healthcare providers. While some aspects of pregnancy may be routine, individual circumstances can vary, necessitating the need for professional guidance. Here are instances when seeking advice from healthcare professionals is crucial:

1. Confirmation of Pregnancy: Scheduling an early appointment with an obstetrician or midwife for confirmation of pregnancy is a fundamental step. This allows healthcare professionals to assess the overall health of the mother and initiate appropriate prenatal care.

2. High-Risk Factors: If there are pre-existing health conditions such as diabetes, hypertension, or a history of complications in previous pregnancies, seeking early and regular consultations becomes essential. High-risk pregnancies often require closer monitoring and specialized care.

3. Medication and Supplement Considerations: Before taking any medications or supplements, including herbal remedies, it's imperative to consult with healthcare professionals. They can provide guidance on the safety and appropriateness of specific interventions during pregnancy.

4. Routine Prenatal Check-ups: Regular prenatal check-ups are a standard component of pregnancy care. These appointments allow healthcare providers to monitor the health of both the mother and the developing baby, address concerns, and provide necessary guidance.

5. Unusual Symptoms or Discomforts: Any unusual symptoms or discomforts, such as severe nausea, persistent headaches, abdominal pain, or changes in fetal movement, should prompt immediate consultation with healthcare professionals. These could be indicative of underlying issues that require attention.

6. Mental Health Concerns: Addressing mental health is an integral part of pregnancy care. If expectant mothers experience symptoms of anxiety, depression, or other mental health challenges, seeking professional advice is crucial. Mental health professionals can offer appropriate support and interventions.

7. Preconception Counseling: For women planning to conceive, preconception counseling provides an opportunity to discuss health history, lifestyle factors, and any concerns with healthcare professionals. This proactive approach helps ensure a healthy start to pregnancy.

8. Birth Plan Discussions: As the due date approaches, discussing and creating a birth plan with healthcare providers is beneficial. This allows expectant mothers to express preferences and understand the available options during labor and delivery.

9. Postpartum Care Planning: Preparing for the postpartum period is an integral part of pregnancy care. Discussing postpartum care plans, including physical recovery, mental health, and breastfeeding support, with healthcare professionals ensures a comprehensive approach to well-being.

Regular communication and collaboration with healthcare professionals create a supportive and informed environment throughout the pregnancy journey. Expectant mothers should feel empowered to raise questions, express concerns, and actively participate in decisions related to their care.

Integrating Herbal Remedies and Aromatherapy with Medical Care

The integration of herbal remedies and aromatherapy with medical care during pregnancy requires careful consideration and collaboration between expectant mothers and healthcare professionals. While these complementary approaches can offer natural support, it's essential to ensure their safety and compatibility with conventional medical practices. Here are insights into integrating herbal remedies and aromatherapy with medical care:

1. Herbal Remedies and Medication Interactions:

Before incorporating herbal remedies, including teas, supplements, or tinctures, it's crucial to consult with healthcare professionals. Some herbs may interact with medications, impacting their efficacy or leading to potential complications.

2. Aromatherapy and Sensitivities:

Essential oils used in aromatherapy can be potent, and individual sensitivities vary. Pregnant women should inform healthcare providers about any planned use of essential oils, especially in the context of labor and delivery. Some hospitals have specific policies regarding aromatherapy.

3. Collaboration with Healthcare Providers:

Open communication with healthcare providers is key when integrating complementary approaches. Sharing details about herbal remedies or aromatherapy practices ensures that professionals are aware of these choices and can offer guidance based on individual health conditions.

4. Safety Considerations:

Certain herbs and essential oils are contraindicated during pregnancy due to potential risks. For example, some herbs may stimulate contractions, and specific essential oils may be too strong for use during pregnancy. Professional advice helps navigate these safety considerations.

5. Individualized Approaches: Healthcare providers can offer individualized guidance based on the unique needs and health status of each expectant mother. This ensures that any integrated herbal or aromatherapy practices align with the overall care plan and well-being goals.

6. Addressing Pregnancy-Related Symptoms: Herbal remedies and aromatherapy can be valuable for addressing

common pregnancy-related symptoms, such as nausea, insomnia, or stress. Collaborating with healthcare providers allows for tailored solutions that complement conventional medical care.

7. Labor and Delivery Preferences: Integrating aromatherapy into labor and delivery preferences should be discussed with healthcare providers and the birthing team. Some hospitals may have policies regarding scents, and ensuring compatibility with the birthing environment is important.

8. Postpartum Support:
Herbal remedies and aromatherapy can also play a role in postpartum support. Discussing these options with healthcare providers allows for a cohesive approach to well-being during the postpartum period.

It's essential to approach the integration of herbal remedies and aromatherapy with a mindset of collaboration and transparency. Healthcare professionals can provide evidence-based guidance, ensuring that these complementary approaches enhance rather than compromise the overall care plan.

Consulting with healthcare professionals is a cornerstone of a healthy and safe pregnancy journey. From routine prenatal check-ups to addressing specific concerns and integrating complementary approaches, the guidance of healthcare providers ensures a comprehensive and individualized approach to care. By fostering open communication and collaboration, expectant mothers can navigate the complexities of pregnancy with confidence and support from their healthcare team.

Self-Appreciation **Notes**

Addressing Common Questions and Concerns

Q1: Is it safe to use herbal remedies and aromatherapy during pregnancy?

Answer: While some herbal remedies and aromatherapy practices can be safe during pregnancy, it's crucial to exercise caution and seek professional advice. Consult with healthcare professionals before using any herbs or essential oils to ensure they are suitable for your specific circumstances. Some substances may have contraindications or potential risks during pregnancy.

Q2: What are common discomforts during pregnancy, and how can herbal remedies help?

Answer: Common discomforts during pregnancy include nausea, fatigue, and muscle aches. Herbal remedies such as ginger for nausea, chamomile for relaxation, and lavender for muscle tension can be beneficial. However, always consult with healthcare providers to ensure safety and appropriateness for your situation.

Q3: How can I maintain a balanced diet during pregnancy?

Answer: Maintaining a balanced diet during pregnancy involves incorporating a variety of nutrient-dense foods. Include fruits, vegetables, whole grains, lean proteins, and dairy products. Consult with a nutritionist or healthcare professional to tailor dietary choices to your specific needs and preferences.

Q4: Are there specific exercises I should avoid during pregnancy?**

Answer: While staying active is important, some exercises may need modification or avoidance during pregnancy. High-impact activities or those with a risk of falls should be approached with caution. Consult with healthcare professionals or prenatal fitness experts for guidance on suitable exercises for your individual circumstances.

Q5: How can I manage stress and anxiety during pregnancy?**

Answer: Managing stress during pregnancy is crucial for both maternal and fetal well-being. Techniques such as mindful breathing, meditation, gentle exercise, and seeking support from friends, family, or mental health professionals can be effective. Always communicate with healthcare providers about your mental health concerns.

Q6: What should I include in my birth plan, and when should I discuss it with my healthcare provider?**

Answer: A birth plan outlines preferences for labor and delivery. Discuss your birth plan with healthcare providers during prenatal visits, ensuring they are aware of your preferences.

Include details such as pain management preferences, birthing environment desires, and any specific considerations you have for the postpartum period.

Q7: Can I continue to use essential oils during labor?**

Answer: The use of essential oils during labor depends on individual preferences, hospital policies, and any potential sensitivities. Discuss your desire to use essential oils during labor with your healthcare provider and the birthing team. Choose mild and well-tolerated scents, and ensure proper ventilation in the birthing environment.

Q8: How can I prepare for the postpartum period?**

Answer: Preparing for the postpartum period involves considering physical and emotional well-being. Discuss postpartum care plans with healthcare providers, including support for breastfeeding, mental health considerations, and physical recovery strategies. Create a support network and communicate openly about your needs and expectations.

Q9: Are there any warning signs during pregnancy that require immediate attention?**

Answer: Certain symptoms during pregnancy may be warning signs, and immediate attention is necessary. These include severe abdominal pain, persistent headaches, changes in fetal movement, or any signs of preterm labor. If you experience unusual symptoms, contact healthcare professionals promptly.

Q10: How can I involve my partner or support system in the pregnancy journey?**

Answer: Involving your partner or support system in the pregnancy journey is valuable. Attend prenatal classes together, communicate openly about expectations, and invite your partner to prenatal appointments. Share your thoughts and feelings, allowing them to be an active part of the experience.

Remember, every pregnancy is unique, Always consult with healthcare professionals for personalized advice and guidance tailored to your specific needs and concerns. Open communication with your healthcare team ensures a supportive and informed approach to navigating the intricacies of pregnancy.

Encouragements for a Healthy and Holistic Pregnancy

Embarking on the journey of pregnancy is a transformative and deeply personal experience. Throughout this guide, we've explored various facets of nurturing a healthy and holistic pregnancy, encompassing herbal remedies, aromatherapy, nutrition, exercise, self-care, and the importance of consulting with healthcare professionals. As we conclude, let's offer encouragement and reflections for expectant mothers on this remarkable journey.

Pregnancy is not merely a physical process; it is a profound and multifaceted transformation that encompasses the physical, emotional, and spiritual dimensions of a woman's life. It is a time of anticipation, growth, and connection – with oneself, one's partner, and the precious life developing within.

Nurturing Holistic Well-being:

A holistic approach to pregnancy involves recognizing the interconnectedness of the mind, body, and spirit. As you navigate the various aspects of herbal remedies, aromatherapy, nutrition, and self-care, remember that your well-being extends beyond the physical realm. Embrace practices that nurture emotional resilience, foster mental calmness, and cultivate a sense of inner balance.

Celebrating Individual Journeys:

Every pregnancy is unique, and so is every woman's journey through it. It's essential to celebrate the individuality of your experience. Your choices, preferences, and feelings are valid and deserve acknowledgment. Whether you find solace in herbal teas, take comfort in aromatherapy, or discover joy in gentle exercises, let your journey unfold in a way that feels authentic and meaningful to you.

The Power of Self-Care:

Self-care is not a luxury but a vital aspect of a healthy pregnancy. It involves intentional practices that honor your well-being. As you engage in herbal remedies, savor aromatherapy moments, and embrace nutritious choices, recognize the power of these acts in contributing to your overall health. Prioritize self-care as an investment in both your own vitality and the well-being of your unborn child.

Partnering with Healthcare Professionals:

The partnership between expectant mothers and healthcare professionals is a cornerstone of a safe and informed pregnancy. Regular consultations, open communication, and collaborative decision-making ensure that your care plan is tailored to your unique needs. Trust the expertise of your healthcare team, and feel empowered to voice your questions and concerns throughout the journey.

A Journey of Growth and Connection:
Pregnancy is not just about the destination of childbirth; it's a profound journey of growth and connection. Embrace the changes, both physical and emotional, as opportunities for self-discovery and resilience. Connect with your partner, your support system, and the broader community of expectant mothers. Share your experiences, offer support, and find strength in the shared journey of bringing new life into the world.

Encouragement for Every Step:
As you take each step on this remarkable journey, let encouragement be your constant companion. Embrace the moments of joy, navigate the challenges with resilience, and remember that you are creating the foundation for a healthy and thriving future. Whether you find solace in the simplicity of a herbal tea, the soothing aroma of essential oils, or the embrace of a supportive community, know that you are not alone.

In conclusion, may this guide serve as a source of inspiration, guidance, and encouragement for a healthy and holistic pregnancy. Cherish the moments, honor your unique path, and trust in the innate strength that accompanies the miracle of bringing life into the world. Wishing you a journey filled with vitality, connection, and the beauty of new beginnings.

Resources and References

Recommended Books and Websites

For further exploration of herbal remedies and aromatherapy during pregnancy, consider the following recommended books and websites:

Books:

1. *The Natural Pregnancy Book: Herbs, Nutrition, and Other Holistic Choices . by Aviva Jill Romm - A comprehensive guide to natural approaches during pregnancy, including herbal remedies.*

2. *Expecting Better: Why the Conventional Pregnancy Wisdom is Wrong and What You Really Need to Know. by Emily Oster - Offers evidence-based insights into various aspects*

of pregnancy, helping you make informed choices.

3. *The Complete Book of Essential Oils and Aromatherapy by Valerie Ann Worwood* - A comprehensive resource on essential oils and aromatherapy, including safety guidelines during pregnancy.

Websites:

1. [American Pregnancy Association](https://americanpregnancy.org/) - Provides information on various aspects of pregnancy, including nutrition, exercise, and wellness.

2. [Herbs for Kids and Pregnancy](https://www.americanherbalistsguild.com/kids-and-pregnancy) - A resource from the American Herbalists Guild offering insights into the safe use of herbs during pregnancy and for children.

3.
[PubMed](https://pubmed.ncbi.nlm.nih.gov/) - A database of scientific studies and research articles. Search for specific topics related to herbal remedies and aromatherapy during pregnancy for in-depth scientific information.

References for Scientific Studies

For a more scientific understanding of herbal remedies and aromatherapy during pregnancy, refer to the following references:

1. Ernst, E. (2002). Herbal medicinal products during pregnancy: are they safe?. BJOG: An International Journal of Obstetrics & Gynaecology, 109(3), 227-235.

2. Smith, C. A., & Collins, C. T. (2016). Crowther, C. A., Crowther, C. A., & Crowther, C. A. (Eds.). Acupuncture or acupressure for pain management during labour. Cochrane Database of Systematic Reviews, 2011(7).

3. Tiran, D. (2010). *Ginger to reduce nausea and vomiting during pregnancy: evidence of effectiveness is not the same as proof of safety.* Complementary Therapies in Clinical Practice, 16(2), 97-100.

4. Davis, M., & Stone, J. (2009). *Understanding aromatherapy.* Journal of Midwifery & Women's Health, 54(5), 377-388.

These references offer a blend of practical advice and evidence-based information, providing a solid foundation for making informed choices during pregnancy. Always consult with healthcare professionals before incorporating new practices into your pregnancy journey.

87 Herbal Remedies And Aromatherapy For A Radiant Pregnancy